Notes on Clinical Information

The Department of Psychiatry Teaching Committee
The Institute of Psychiatry, London

LONDON
OXFORD UNIVERSITY PRESS
NEW YORK   TORONTO

Oxford University Press, Ely House, London W.1

*Glasgow New York Toronto Melbourne Wellington
Cape Town Ibadan Nairobi Dar es Salaam Lusaka Addis Ababa
Delhi Bombay Calcutta Madras Karachi Lahore Dacca
Kuala Lumpur Singapore Hong Kong Tokyo*

ISBN 0 19 264166 2

©Oxford University Press 1973

*First published 1973
Reprinted 1975*

All rights reserved. No part of this publication may be reproduced, stored in a retrieval system, or transmitted, in any form or by any means, electronic, mechanical, photocopying, recording or otherwise, without the prior permission of Oxford University Press.

This book is sold subject to the condition that it shall not, by way of trade or otherwise, be lent, re-sold, hired out, or otherwise circulated without the publisher's prior consent in any form of binding or cover other than that in which it is published and without a similar condition including this condition being imposed on the subsequent purchaser.

Contents

Preface	vii
Introduction	1
Psychiatric Interviewing	1
The History	3
The Psychiatric Examination (Mental State)	8
The Summary	12
Formulations	13
Progress Notes	14

Appendices

A.	Further Examination of Patients with Suspected Organic Cerebral Disease	14
B.	Examination of the Mute or Apparently Inaccessible Patient	20
C.	The Gresham Ward Questionnaires	22

Preface

These notes on the eliciting and recording of clinical information were drawn up by the Teaching Committee of the Department of Psychiatry, primarily for the use of registrars in the Maudsley and Bethlem Royal Hospitals. They are intended to provide guidance for those with little previous experience of psychiatry on the scope and organization of psychiatric case notes and also to ensure that a fairly uniform style and layout are used for the recording of clinical data throughout the Joint Hospital.

These notes replace the earlier Notes on Casetaking which have now been in use unchanged for over twenty years. Although the general style and format is much the same in both documents there are several changes of emphasis. New sections have been introduced into the History for adolescence and drug abuse, for example, in recognition of their increasing importance in contemporary psychiatric practice; and several of the cognitive tests in the original mental state examination have been omitted because of the evidence we now have that they discriminate poorly between patients with organic and functional disturbances. The document as a whole is also considerably longer than its predecessor. This should not be taken to imply a belief on our part that case notes should be more comprehensive than they have been in the past; but it does reflect our belief that the eliciting and recording of information are matters of fundamental importance to all clinical psychiatrists and that as much guidance as possible should be given in these skills.

There are two main sections, the first concerned with the History and the second with the Psychiatric Examination or Mental State. There are other sections also dealing with psychiatric interviewing in general and with progress notes and summaries, and appendices containing detailed schemata for the examination of patients who are mute or are suspected of having organic cerebral disease.

Many people have contributed to these notes, and we would like to take this opportunity of thanking those members of the hospital staff — consultants, senior registrars and registrars — who read through the early drafts and tried them out in practice. Their advice and comments were invaluable and led to several important changes. In particular we would like to thank Professor David Marsden and Dr Frank Benson for their expert help in the preparation of the section on the examination of patients with organic cerebral disease.

The Institute of Psychiatry,	D. Hill (Chairman)	
de Crespigny Park,	J.L.T. Birley	F. Post
London, S.E.5.	R.H. Cawley	M.L. Rutter
July, 1972.	R.E. Kendell	J.K. Wing
	W.A. Lishman	H.H. Wolff

Introduction

This document sets out the principles which should be followed when compiling the medical notes of patients in the Joint Hospital. A high standard of clinical recording is a hallmark of good medical practice and is nowhere more important than in psychiatry. The situation is more complex here than in other fields of medicine because so many different types of information are relevant to the evaluation and management of clinical problems. Many disciplines are involved in psychiatry and there are several contrasting approaches both to theoretical and practical issues. For this reason there can be no final and comprehensive statement about clinical methods which would apply to all patients in all situations, and which would be regarded as appropriate by all experienced clinicians. Differences of emphasis are to be found in different units in the Joint Hospital. The notes which follow should be regarded as a set of general principles which call for flexibility in their application. Registrars will find it necessary to be selective and to introduce variations to meet the needs of particular patients and of specialized departments. In the Out-Patient Department, for example, a considerably abbreviated scheme is required for both eliciting and recording clinical information, though the principles remain unchanged.

Psychiatric Interviewing

The examination of a psychiatric patient resembles a general medical examination in many respects, but there are important differences. These derive partly from the fact that in psychiatry much more attention needs to be paid to psychological and social phenomena, but the main difference arises from the fact that it is the interview itself which serves as the psychiatrist's main tool of investigation.

Psychiatric interviewing is thus a specialized technique of great importance. Three aspects may be distinguished; in different contexts each may assume prime importance but skilled interviewing aims at incorporating all three whenever possible:

1. The interview is a technique for obtaining information. Its objective is to obtain as accurate an account as possible of the patient's illness, the facts of his background and the significant events in his life, and to gain some understanding of his experiences and his attitudes towards a variety of people and circumstances. To these ends the examiner must have a clear idea of the range of information he wants, so that he can guide the interview from one subject to another until he is satisfied that everything has been covered. The flow of the interview depends on what the patient says, but the examiner is in control. Nonetheless even here it is important to be ready to listen to what the patient wants to say, even if this means putting off certain important questions until later. Questions must be framed in a form which the patient readily understands, and presented with tact and sensitivity.

2. The interview also serves as a standard situation in which to assess the patient's emotions and attitudes. If the interview is to be effective for this purpose, 'wooden' or stereotyped questioning must be avoided, and the examiner must be warm, empathic and responsive. He needs to be alert to the implications of the patient's facial expression, his tone of voice, his comments and his gestures. During the course of the interview, even when discussing relatively straightforward topics, the patient will give many clues about the sort of person he is and his attitudes and reactions to others (including the interviewer). The examiner should also be able, from his own reactions to the patient, to gain further useful information about him. In fact, the total interaction between doctor and patient is a most important source of information about the patient's personality and mental state, and this interaction should be observed and described by the physician, who with experience learns to do so more objectively and skilfully.

3. The interview, and especially the first interview, fulfils in addition a valuable supportive role and serves to establish an understanding with the patient which will be the basis of the subsequent working relationship. Comments which make the patient realize he is being understood are likely to increase his confidence, while too rigid an insistence on a predetermined form of questioning or ill-timed interruptions will have the reverse effect. In the case of many anxious, suspicious or hostile patients, the factual detail obtainable at the first interview may need to be limited. Patient empathic listening is particularly important in such cases and the patient should not be hurried or pressed for answers to questions which he may at first consider irrelevant or embarrassing. Several

interviews may be necessary to obtain anything like a complete picture. Anxiety to achieve this too quickly may not only impede the process but also undermine the relationship on which future interviews and treatment are to be based.

It is important to distinguish between the manner in which information is obtained and the way in which it is subsequently recorded. It is therefore important to retain in one's mind what is ultimately required for a complete history, and at the same time to approach each interview in the light of the patient's present needs.

The *history* will record data obtained from several sources; it is concerned with the patient's complaints, his recent and remote past, and his present life situation up to the time of admission (or referral in the case of an out-patient). The *examination of the mental state* is concerned with verbal and non-verbal behaviour systematically observed during the interview. Additional observations made elsewhere, either on the ward or in other parts of the hospital, should be recorded under the latter heading, stating their source (informant).

History

The history should be compiled from information elicited both from the patient and from one or more informants. Only in exceptional circumstances should the informant be interviewed before the patient is himself seen. The informant's account will not only amplify the patient's reports of factual detail but also shed light on the patient's relationships within and without the family. Information from the patient and from different informants should be kept distinct *and recorded on separate sheets*. Specify the informant's name, relationship to the patient, intimacy and length of acquaintance. Also record your impression of the informant's reliability and his attitudes to the patient and to the illness. (It may also be important to record the names, addresses and telephone numbers of other potential informants.)

The following areas of information should be covered in every case, although details recorded under each heading may vary with individual circumstances. The order in which these various topics are listed is the order in which they should appear in the clinical notes, but it may be appropriate to arrange them differently when obtaining the information in the first place, or when reading the case history to someone who is unfamiliar with it. In this latter case it is often helpful to give a brief 'thumbnail sketch' — two or three sentences — before embarking on the detailed presentation.

Reason for Referral

Brief statement of why and how the patient came to hospital.

Complaints

Reported by patient, in his own words, not limited to main complaints, and the duration of each complaint.

Present Illness

A detailed account of the illness from the earliest time at which a change was noted until admission to hospital. The sequence of various symptoms should be dated approximately. Note the life situation and the patient's reaction to it at all relevant times in the course of the illness. State previous treatment of present illness and its effects.

Associated Impairments: describe changes in the patient's relationships with people in marriage, social and sexual life and work; alteration in sleep, eating, weight, excretory functions and drinking and smoking habits; and changes in his capacity for making decisions, taking responsibilities and communicating with others.

Family History

(In cases of fostering, adoption, step-parents, etc. the record should include data concerning the biological and the social family.)
Mother: age, or age and patient's age at the time of her death, and cause of death. Occupation. Mental and physical illnesses; personality. Patient's relationship to her in childhood and subsequently, and reaction to her death. Periods of separation in childhood: duration and circumstances.
Father: data as for Mother. Always record details of his occupation.
Sibs: enumerate in chronological order of birth, with first names, ages, marital state, occupation, significant illnesses, personality. (Include miscarriages and stillbirths.) Patient's previous and current relationship with them.
Other relatives: familial diseases, alcoholism, abnormal personalities, mental disorder, epilepsy (say so if information is lacking). Note the place and time of psychiatric treatment received by members of family.

Family atmosphere in childhood: salient happenings affecting parents and collaterals during patient's early years. Emotional relationships within the family. Early stresses arising from emotional or economic causes, including death of, or separation from, close relatives, and patient's age at the time.

Personal History

Early development: date and place of birth, birth weight. Abnormalities during pregnancy and childbirth. Feeding difficulties. Delicate or healthy baby. Precocious or retarded, e.g. in talking and walking. Habit training difficulties. Mother's attitude towards early development.

Behaviour during childhood: persistent sleep difficulties, bedwetting, stammering, tics or mannerisms. Recurrent abdominal pains, fears, periods of misery, shyness, excessive conformity. Hyperactivity, serious mischief, frequent fights, truancy, delinquency. Play activities and make-believe. Ability to make and keep friendships. Attitudes to sibs, parents and strangers and response to birth of sibs, separation from parents, and to other family crises and bereavements.

School: age of beginning and finishing. Types of schools. Examinations passed or failed. Prolonged absences from school; years repeated; specific difficulties, e.g. reading. Bullied or teased. Attitude to peers, teachers and work.

Occupations: age of starting work. Jobs held, in chronological order, and reasons for change. Satisfaction in work or reasons for dissatisfaction. Competence. Ambition and prospects. Relationship with others at work. Detailed inquiry into war experiences and disabilities. Promotion in Forces. Stability under stress.

Adolescence: attitude to growing up, to peers, to family, to authority. Rebelliousness. Drug-taking. Periods of depression or withdrawal. Fantasy life.

Sexual history: age at onset of puberty (voice-breaking, shaving, menarche); how regarded. Masturbation: age, fantasies and anxieties. Homosexual and heterosexual fantasies, inclinations and experiences, apart from marriage. Sexual disorders, impotence, frigidity, and other difficulties. Describe any deviations. Current sexual practice – marital and extra-marital. Contraception. Sexual satisfaction, dissatisfaction and anxieties.

Marital history: number of previous engagements, associated circumstances. Duration of courtship. Age at marriage (or marriages). Age, occupation, health (past and present) and personality of marital partner. Marital relationship and problems in the past and at present. Marriage forced by pregnancy. Fidelity of partners.

Where applicable, dates of deaths of spouses, divorces or separations.
Children: chronological list of pregnancies (including spontaneous and induced abortions). Ages and names of children, their physical and mental health in the past and at present time. State place and time of psychiatric treatment received by children. Attitudes towards children and further pregnancies.

Medical History: (a) *Health during childhood*: deliria, chorea, fits, periods of unconsciousness from any cause; (b) *Menstrual history*: regularity, pain, duration, abnormalities. Emotional disturbance. Date of last period. Menopausal symptoms; (c) *General*: illnesses, operations, head injuries, accidents, hospitalizations in chronological order. Patient's reactions to these.

Previous mental health: details of all psychiatric conditions for which treatment has been received, giving dates and duration of illness, and nature of treatment. Specify names of hospitals and doctors.

Details of all psychiatric disturbances for which treatment has *not* been received (e.g. behaviour disturbances, alcohol or drug abuse, preoccupation with bodily functions, insomnia, mood variations, psychophysiological disturbances, anxiety symptoms, etc.). Describe in each case the life situation which prevailed at the time.

Use and abuse of alcohol, tobacco and drugs: smoking and drinking habits, including an estimate of the quantities involved recently, and also in the past if significantly different then. Attempts to give up and their success. Evidence of effects on health, relationships with others, ability to work effectively, and finances. Any use of cannabis, LSD, amphetamines or heroin. Excessive use of aspirin, etc. Dependence on hypnotics or tranquillizers, whether obtained on prescription or not.

Antisocial behaviour: delinquency or criminal offences, even if never convicted. Periods in prison, Borstal, remand home, etc. or on probation. Any history of violence or assault. Excessive gambling.

Life situation at present: description of patient's family, housing, social, work and financial circumstances. Satisfactions and dissatisfactions with these. Composition of household. Difficulties with neighbours. Other significant relationships and patient's attitudes towards them. Evidence of emotional conflict in family, sexual or work relationships; recent stresses, bereavements, losses or disappointments and the patient's reactions to them.

Personality

The personality of a patient consists of those habitual attitudes and patterns of behaviour, which together with his physical characteristics distinguish him as an individual to others and to himself. Personality sometimes changes after the onset of a mental illness. *If so, what is wanted here is a description of his personality before the illness began. This will require information from other informants as well as the patient himself.* Some of the relevant information will have been recorded under the various headings in the personal history − e.g. how the patient has behaved in different social roles − as a child, parent, sibling, spouse, employee, etc. Other areas of personality functioning are indicated below. Aim to build up a picture of an individual, not a type. Do not merely give a list of adjectives and epithets, which are given here only as guide-lines. *Consider the seven headings listed below and using the data elicited write a one- or two-paragraph description of the patient's personality in non-technical language.*

1. **Attitudes to others in social, family and sexual relationships**: ability to trust others and make and sustain relationships; anxious or secure, leader or follower. Participation, responsibility, capacity to make decisions. Friendly, warm, demonstrative, reserved, cold, indifferent. Secretive, competitive, jealous. Dominant, submissive, ambivalent. Authoritarian, dependent. Aggressive, quarrelsome, sensitive, suspicious, resentful. Different attitudes to own and opposite sex. Evidence of difficulty in role-taking − gender, sexual, familial, parental and work.

2. **Attitudes to self**: egocentric, selfish, indulgent. Vain, self-dramatizing. Critical, deprecatory. Overconcerned, self-conscious. Attitudes to own performance in different roles. Satisfaction or dissatisfaction with self. Ambition. Attitudes to own health, bodily functions; over-concerned, neglectful. Realistic or unrealistic self-appraisal. Attitudes to past achievements and failures, to the future and to dying.

3. **Moral and religious attitudes and standards**: rigid, uncompromising, compliant. Easy, permissive, over-conscientious, perfectionist. Conforming, rebellious. Religious beliefs.

4. **Mood**: stable, changeable, swings of mood. Optimistic, pessimistic. Anxious, irritable, worrying, tense. Lively, apathetic. Ability to express and control feelings of anger, sadness, pleasure, disappointment, etc. Inhibited, open.

5. **Leisure activities and interests**: books, plays, pictures, music, etc. preferred. Sport and other leisure activities. Creative activities. Spends leisure time alone, with one or two friends or many friends.

6. **Fantasy life**: day dreams, dreams and nightmares.

7. **Reaction pattern to stress**: (in suitable cases a life-chart should be drawn up). Ability to tolerate frustration, losses, disappointments, and circumstances arousing anger, anxiety or depression. Evidence

for the excessive use of particular defence mechanisms such as denial, rationalization, projection, etc. Evidence of intellectual, educational or emotional deficits in the personality incompatible with roles the patient is called upon to take. Evidence for inadequate gratification of biological or social needs through life circumstances or personality inadequacy or deviation.

The Psychiatric Examination (Mental State)

The description of the patient's mental state should record behavioural and psychological data elicited by examination at the time of the interview as well as observations made in the ward and other parts of the hospital. It has already been pointed out that there are three aspects to interviewing — obtaining information, observing the patient in a two-person interaction, and giving support. The areas of information that need to be covered in the 'mental state' examination are detailed below. The opportunity should also be taken to record the way the patient reacts to the interviewer and how the interviewer himself feels.

1. **Appearance and general behaviour**: description as complete, accurate and lifelike as possible of how the patient appears and what can be observed in his behaviour. Way of spending the day, eating, sleep, cleanliness in general, self-care, hair, cosmetics, dress. Behaviour towards other patients, doctors and nursing staff. Is the patient relaxed or tense and restless? Slow, hesitant, repetitive? Do movements and attitudes have an apparent purpose or meaning? How does he respond to various requirements and situations? Are there abnormal responses to external events? Can his attention be held, and diverted?

Does the patient's behaviour suggest that he is disoriented? Specify orientation if doubtful. Describe gestures, grimaces, and other motor expressions. Is there much or little activity? Does it vary in the day, spontaneous or how provoked? Does he, if inactive, resist passive movements or maintain an attitude or obey commands or indicate awareness at all? Do hallucinations seem to modify behaviour? Even if the patient does not speak, there should still be a full and careful report of his posture and behaviour.

2. **Talk**: the *form* of the patient's utterances rather than their content is here considered. Does he say much or little, talk

spontaneously or only in answer, slowly or quickly, hesitantly or promptly, to the point or wide of it, coherently, anxiously, discursively, loosely with interruptions, with sudden silences, with frequent changes of topic, commenting on events and things at hand, appropriately, using strange words or syntax, rhymes, puns? How does the form of his talk vary with its subject? Attach or include in the notes any abnormal written productions. A verbatim sample of talk should be recorded at this point if there are abnormalities of form. It should give an adequate demonstration of formal disorders of thinking such as flight of ideas, thought block, disorders of association, reiterations, perseveration, incoherence, neologisms, paraphasias, etc.

3. **Mood**: the patient's appearance, motility, posture and general behaviour as already described above may give some indication of his mood. In addition, his answers to questions such as 'how do you feel in yourself?', 'what is your mood?', 'how about your spirits?' or some similar inquiry should be recorded. Ask about suicidal thoughts and attitudes to the future whenever depressive mood is suspected. Many varieties of mood may be present, not merely happiness or sadness, i.e. such states as anxiety, fear, suspicion, perplexity and others which it is convenient to include under this heading. Observe the constancy of the mood during the interview, the influences which change it and the appropriateness of the patient's apparent emotional state to what he says. Note evidence of flatness or lability of affect and specify any indications that the patient is concealing his true feelings.

4. **Thought content**: this should include morbid thoughts and preoccupations. The patient's answers to questions such as 'what do you see as your main worries' should be summarized. Are there anxieties or preoccupations with the present life situation, with the future, with the past, with the safety of the self or others? Do worries interfere with concentration or sleep? Phobias or obsessional ruminations, compulsions, or rituals. Suicidal thoughts, wishes, fears or plans.

5. **Abnormal beliefs and interpretations of events**: specify the content, mode of onset and degree of fixity of any abnormal beliefs:
- (a) in relation to the environment, e.g. ideas of reference, misinterpretations or delusions. Beliefs that he is being persecuted, that he is being treated in a special way, or is the subject of an experiment;
- (b) in relation to the body, e.g. ideas or delusions of bodily change;
- (c) in relation to the self, e.g. delusions of passivity, influence, thought reading or intrusion.

6. **Abnormal experiences referred to environment, body or self**:
    (a) to the environment (e.g. hallucinations and illusions — auditory, visual, olfactory, gustatory or tactile; feelings of familiarity or unfamiliarity; derealization; *déjà-vu*);
    (b) to the body (e.g. feelings of deadness, pain or other alterations of bodily sensation, somatic hallucinations);
    (c) to the self (e.g. depersonalization, awareness of disturbance in mechanism of thinking, or blocking, or retardation, autochthonous ideas, etc.)

The source, content, vividness, reality and other characteristics of these experiences should be recorded, and also the time of occurrence, e.g. at night, when alone, when falling asleep or awakening.

7. **The cognitive state**: this should be briefly assessed in every patient and related to his general intelligence (see under *Intelligence*). In younger patients who are not suspected of cerebral organic disease, the tests mentioned in the following notes for orientation, attention, concentration and memory should be administered. In older patients the Gresham Ward questionnaires* of orientation, past and recent memory, and general information may be given and copies should be available on every ward. A low score (less than about thirty-five points), patchiness or perseveration should lead to further inquiry.

When cognitive impairment or cerebral disease is suspected, further tests will need to be given from the schema for 'Further examination of patients with suspected organic cerebral disease'. (Appendix A)

Orientation: if there is any reason to doubt the patient's orientation, record the patient's answers to questions about his own name and identity, the place where he is, the time of day, the date.

Attention and Concentration: is his attention easily aroused and sustained? Does he concentrate? Is he easily distracted? To test his concentration and attention, ask him to tell the days or the months in reverse order, or to do simple arithmetical problems requiring 'carrying over' (e.g. 112-25) or subtraction of serial 7s from 100 (give answers and time taken). Give digits to repeat forwards, and then others to repeat backwards (delivered evenly and at one second intervals) and record how many he can reproduce.

Memory: in all cases memory should be assessed by comparing the patient's account of his life with that given by others, and by examining his account for intrinsic evidence of gaps or in-

*See Appendix C or Post, F. (1965) *The Clinical Psychiatry of Late Life*, pp. 33-34 and 47-51, Oxford.

consistencies. Special attention should be paid to memory for recent events such as those of his admission to hospital and happenings in the ward since. Where there is selective impairment of memory for special incidents, periods, recent or remote happenings, this should be recorded in detail, and the patient's attitude to his forgetfulness and the things forgotten especially investigated. Record any evidence of confabulation or false memories. If the patient confabulates, is this spontaneous or in response to suggestion only? Retrograde and anterograde amnesia must be specified in detail in relation to head injury or epileptic phenomena.

If there is any suspicion of impairment of memory, record verbatim the patient's attempt to repeat a name and address or other similar data, immediately and five minutes later. Test ability to repeat immediately after a single hearing a Stanford-Binet sentence appropriate to the patient's intellectual level.* Test the number of repetitions necessary for accurate reproduction of one of the Babcock sentences.**

Intelligence: the patient's expected intelligence should be gauged from his history, his general knowledge, his educational and occupational record. Where this is unknown simple tests for general information and grasp should be given and an assessment made of his experience and interests. In general, every patient should complete the Mill Hill and Progressive Matrices tests and results should be recorded here. If there are discrepancies in the results between these tests and the anticipated intelligence, try to interpret them.

8. **Patient's appraisal of illness, difficulties and prospects**: what is the patient's attitude to his present state? Does he regard it as an illness, as 'physical', 'mental' or 'nervous', as needing treatment? What does he attribute it to? Is he aware of mistakes made spontaneously or in response to tests? How does he regard them and other details of his condition? How does he regard previous experiences, mental illnesses, etc.? Can he appreciate possible connexions between his illness and stressful life situations, spontaneously or when suggested? Are his attitudes constructive or

---

*(e.g. Year 11: 'Yesterday we went for a ride in our car along the road that crosses the bridge.' Year 13: 'The aeroplane made a careful landing in the space which had been prepared for it'. Average adult: 'The red-headed woodpeckers made a terrible fuss as they tried to drive the young away from the nest'. Superior adult: 'At the end of the week, the newspaper published a complete account of the experiences of the great explorer'.

**(e.g. 'The one thing a nation needs in order to be rich and great is a large secure supply of wood', or 'The clouds hung low in the valley and the wind howled among the trees as the men went on through the rain'.)

unconstructive, realistic or unrealistic? Is his judgement good when discussing financial, domestic problems, etc.? What does he propose to do when he has left the hospital?

9. **The interviewer's reaction to the patient**: here a brief account should be given of the way in which the interviewer is affected by the patient's behaviour. Did he make him feel sympathetic, concerned, sad, anxious, irritated, frustrated, impatient or angry? Did the interviewer find it easy or difficult to control any untoward responses evoked in him, or has he failed to do so and, if so, how?

The Summary

This is an important document which should be drawn up with care. Its purpose is to provide a concise description of all the important aspects of the case, to enable others who are unfamiliar with the patient to grasp the essential features of the problem without needing to search elsewhere for further information.

The first part should be completed within 2 weeks of admission and be drawn up under the following headings:

Reason for Referral
Complaint (or complaints)
Present Illness
Family History
Personal History
    Childhood
    Occupations
    Marriage and children
    Personality
    Physical health
    Previous mental health
Physical Examination
Psychiatric Examination

The summary of the Psychiatric Examination should cover all important aspects of the mental state, positive and negative, and be drawn up under whichever of the sub-headings in the main schema are necessary to achieve this. The six sub-headings of Personal History listed above should always be included, and others from the main schema introduced as appropriate.

The second part should be completed within 1 week of discharge and be laid out under the following headings:

Investigations
Treatment and Progress
Final Diagnosis (or diagnoses) and amplifying comment
Prognosis (make a predictive statement related to symptoms and social adaptation, rather than terms like guarded, good or poor)
Condition on Discharge
Further Management

The completed summary should be short enough to go on two sides of A4 paper when typed, but only rarely so short that it does not cover one side.

The summary of a readmission should include the full range of categories listed here, unless the last admission was very recent and it has been established that no significant change has occurred in the family history and personal history in the interim.

References to highly confidential matters (criminal acts, sexual revelations, etc.) should only be included if their omission would produce serious distortion of the over-all picture. Often it will be preferable to include only a veiled reference followed by 'see notes' in brackets.

Formulations

Initial Formulation

After completing the mental state and history a 'formulation' should be composed, on a separate sheet. This is the registrar's own assessment of the case rather than a restatement of the facts, and its length, layout and emphasis will vary considerably from one patient to another. It should always include a discussion of the diagnosis, of the aetiological factors which seem important, taking into account the patient's life situation and background, a plan of treatment and an estimate of prognosis. Regardless of the uncertainty or complexity of the case a provisional diagnosis should always be specified, using the nomenclature of the International Classification and the glossary to this.

Final Formulation

This is a revision of the initial formulation drawn up at the time of discharge. It should specify any divergencies of opinion and should state the views of the consultant clearly. It should be written in the light of the patient's response to treatment and other information becoming available since the time of admission. As before, its length and layout will vary considerably, but it should always include a final diagnosis, with amplifying comments, and an estimate of prognosis.

Progress Notes

Regular progress notes, signed and dated, are a vital part of every case record. They should describe the treatment the patient is receiving (with dates of starting and finishing, and dosages of all drugs), significant changes in mental state and any important events involving the patient. They should also record the opinions expressed by consultants at ward rounds and case conferences. Although these notes must be detailed enough to convey an accurate picture of the patient's treatment and his response to it, they should not normally contain lengthy verbatim accounts of conversations between patient and doctor. Notes which are excessively long are never read.

A *handover note* should be written whenever the patient is transferred from the care of one registrar to another, summarizing the salient features and outlining future plans. This is particularly important in the case of out-patients for whom there is no formal summary or formulation.

Appendix A
Further Examination of Patients With Suspected Organic Cerebral Disease

Patients with specific or general defects of cerebral function may or may not be aware of them, and may or may not be able to direct attention to the disabilities produced by these defects. Examination for such defects should follow a full neurological examination which may direct detailed inquiry to particular functions.

Testing must not be hurried; *the patient may tire easily and several sessions may be needed for complete examination.*

The schema of examination and selection of tests must always be adapted to the needs and difficulties of the individual patient and to his intelligence and educational level. The order in which the tests are offered will often need to be altered when special disabilities emerge. One disability may have important effects on performance at other tasks (e.g. receptive dysphasia on tests of dyspraxia) and due allowance must be made for this in the administration of tests and the assessment of results.

In all cases, however, it is advisable to adhere to a simple routine at the start of the examination:
1. First evaluate the patient's level of conscious awareness.
2. Next decide whether language functions are intact.*
3. Assess the patient's memory, and particularly his ability to store new information.
4. Use simple screening tests for spatial and constructional ability.**

Assessment of consciousness and of language functions is essential at the outset, since the interpretation of other tests will depend upon the patient's ability to co-operate and on the accuracy of verbal communication between patient and examiner. Memory functions deserve attention next because they provide a sensitive index of many forms of cerebral disorder. Screening tests of spatial and constructional ability are necessary because such non-verbal deficits may otherwise remain concealed.

The leads derived from the above, together with the patient's complaints and relatives' observations, will then direct attention to areas which must be studied in greater detail as described below. Finally other functions which have at first sight appeared to be intact should be examined by simple abbreviated tests.

Level of Conscious Awareness

Fluctuations in level of consciousness during testing should be recorded. The relatives or nursing staff should be questioned about changes from time to time during the day, with specific inquiry for diurnal variation.

Evidence suggesting a minor degree of impairment of consciousness may have been obtained from the tests of orientation,

*Language functions can be rapidly assessed by: (a) estimating the patient's verbal ability during conversation and history taking; (b) asking him to name a series of objects; (c) presenting him with a series of written commands to point to specific objects; (d) asking him to write down the names of objects to which you point.

**By asking the patient to execute simple drawings and to copy simple designs selected from those on page 18.

attention, concentration and memory outlined in the general section of the mental state. The possibility that fluctuation in the level of consciousness has interfered with registration of ongoing experience, including that of the interview itself, must be considered. Is the patient alert or dull, wide awake or drowsy? If somnolent, can he be roused to full or only partial awareness? If the patient's attention cannot be sustained does he drift back into sleep or does his attention wander on to other topics? Eyes open or shut, fixed or following movement? State of bladder and bowels? The level of consciousness should be documented by defining the nature of the stimulus required to evoke the response and the character of that response.* Evidence for delirium, stupor or coma should be specified in detail.

Language Function

Motor Aspects of Speech. Note the quality of spontaneous speech and that in response to questions. Is there any disturbance of articulation (dysarthria)? Is there slowness or hesitancy with production? Does he have difficulty finding words, or use circumlocutions? Does he use wrong words, words that do not exist (neologisms), or words which are nearly but not exactly correct (paraphasias)? Are there inaccuracies of grammatical construction (paragrammatisms)? Are words omitted and sentences abbreviated (telegram style)? Is speech totally disorganized and incomprehensible (jargon aphasia)? Observe for perseverative errors of speech, echolalia or palilalia.

Note any discrepancy between what is possible in spontaneous speech, and in reply to questions. Minor expressive speech defects may only emerge when the patient is pressed to engage in conversation, to describe his work, his home, or some event in his life. Test whether automatic speech or the naming of serials is better preserved than conversational speech — ask him to count to twenty, give the days of the week, or repeat a nursery rhyme. Are emotional utterances and ejaculations preserved when formal speech is defective?

---

*Appropriate stimuli in ascending order of intensity are conversation, shouted commands, commands coming after arousal by shaking, moderate pain as produced by pin prick and pain produced by supra-orbital or sternal pressure. The response may be a correct verbal reply or motor act to command, an incorrect verbal reply or motor act, a failure to reply to any command, an incorrect verbal reply or motor act, a failure to reply to any command but accurate manual location of a painful stimulus, or at worst decorticate or decerebrate responses to painful stimuli.

NOTE: From the phenomenological point of view dysphasic speech may be usefully classified into fluent and non-fluent varieties. Fluent dysphasias in general show normal or excessive output, clear articulation, normal or long phrase length, normal rhythm and inflexion, frequent paraphasic errors, and are produced without effort. Non-fluent dysphasias show sparse output, poor articulation, short phrase length, disturbed rhythm and inflexion, meaningful content when this can be discerned, and speech is produced with obvious difficulty.

Comprehension of Speech. The understanding of speech must be assessed separately, whether or not production is defective. Even if the patient is mute or his utterances totally incomprehensible it is still necessary to determine whether he can comprehend what is said to him. Can he point correctly on command to one of several objects displayed to view? Can he signal his response to simple 'yes − no' questions? Can he carry out simple orders on request, e.g. pick up an object, or show his tongue; can he respond to more complex instructions, e.g. walk over to the door and come back again, or take his spectacles from his pocket and put them on the table?

If comprehension of speech is defective, test whether understanding of written words and instructions is better preserved. Test whether other hearing functions are intact (e.g. startle response to noise). Test whether he can recognize non-verbal noises, e.g. clapping hands, snapping fingers, rattling money, or copy the production of such sounds when they are made outside the field of vision (auditory agnosia).

Repetition of Speech. Can the patient repeat digits, words, short phrases or long sentences exactly as you give them? (This involves both motor and sensory parts of the speech apparatus and also the connexions between the two.)

Word Finding. Test specifically for nominal dysphasia by asking the patient to name both common and uncommon objects and colours presented to him. (This may be the only language disturbance in patients with cerebral damage.)

Writing. Can he write spontaneously and to dictation? Are written productions defective (substitutions, perseveration, spelling errors, letter reversals)? Is copying better preserved than writing to dictation? Is spelling out loud better preserved than spelling on paper? Is the writing of habitual material (signature, address) relatively intact? Are numbers written more accurately than words or letters?

Reading. Test ability to read aloud and to perform simple written and printed instructions. Failing this, can he identify single words or letters? Does he comprehend normally what he reads?

Whenever language disturbances are evident, assess the patient's own awareness of them. *Is he predominantly right or left handed?*

Memory Functions

Full examination of memory functions will always be required along the lines set out in the body of the document. Special attention should be directed at recent memory and learning ability. Non-verbal memory should always be tested in addition to verbal memory by asking the patient to reproduce simple figures (see below) after an interval of five minutes.

Visuospatial and Constructional Difficulties

Test the patient's ability to judge the relations between objects in space — to estimate distances, to say which of two objects is nearer to him, which is larger, etc. Can he with eyes closed indicate the spatial order of objects in the room around him?

Visuospatial agnosia is often associated with constructional dyspraxia. Test ability to connect two given dots by a straight line, to find the middle of a straight line or a circle. Test his ability to draw simple figures (square, circle, triangle). Ask him to copy a series of line drawings of increasing complexity such as those shown below, directly and from immediate memory:

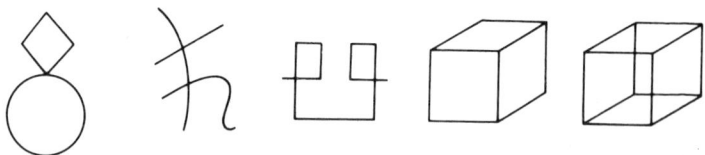

Ask him to draw a house, a clock face and set the hands, to indicate principal towns on a rough map of Great Britain. In such tests and in written productions generally, does he crowd material into a corner of the paper or show unilateral neglect of visual space?

Test ability to construct with sticks or matches a triangle, a square, or to reproduce more complex designs presented to him. Can he assemble a simple jigsaw puzzle or re-assemble a piece of paper cut into fragments? If available, test his ability to reproduce patterns with Koh's blocks.

Visual Agnosia

Can the patient describe what he sees and identify objects and persons? Ask him to name a particular object in a group exposed to view, to describe its use, or if dysphasic to indicate its use. (If he fails, test whether he can identify it by touch.) Ask him to name the colours of objects. Ask him to describe a meaningful situation in a picture shown to him. Is his recognition of faces defective (prosopagnosia)? Ask him to point out a named person known to him among a group, or to name photographs of relatives or well-known public figures.

Dyspraxia

Test the patient's ability to carry out purposeful movements to command, e.g. holding out arms, crossing legs, showing teeth, screwing up eyes, nodding head. Test each hand separately for opening and closing the hand, opposition of thumb and little finger, pronation and supination. Test the patient's ability to carry out complex co-ordinated sequences of movements to command, e.g. light a match, wind a watch, fold paper and put it in an envelope. (Several varieties of dyspraxia are sometimes recognized — limb kinetic, ideomotor, and ideational.)

Other Disturbances of Cortical Function

Number Functions. Can the patient read or write numbers of two and more digits? Can he count objects and guess without counting the number of matches laid before him? Assess ability to handle number concepts — addition, subtraction, multiplication, division — in relation to his educational and occupational background. Assess ability to handle money correctly.

Topographical Disorientation. Does the patient find his way easily about the ward when he would be expected to do so? Does he confuse his bed with other people's? Can he describe the relations between parts of the ward or of his own house, can he describe the route from home to hospital? If necessary test his ability to follow on command a simple route in the ward or hospital.

Right—Left Disorientation. Can he point on command to objects around him on the right and on the left? Ask him to move on command right and left parts of the body, to point to individual parts on the right and on the left side of his own body, and of the examiner sitting opposite him. Can he perform complex instructions like 'touch your right ear with your left hand', 'pick up the left hand match with your left hand and place it in my right hand'?

Body Image Disturbances. These may include:

(i) *Finger Agnosia.* Ask the patient to name, move on command or point to individual fingers — his own and the examiner's.

(ii) *Disturbances of identification of body parts (autotopagnosia).* Ask the patient to move on command and to name various parts of his body, to point to them and to parts of the examiner's body.

(iii) *Unawareness or neglect of body parts (anosognosia).* The patient may ignore an injured or functionally defective part of his body, e.g. hemiplegic limbs or hemianopic field defect. He may verbally deny the functional defect or deny ownership of the affected body part.

Dressing Difficulties. Does the patient show undue difficulty in dressing and undressing, get muddled when inserting limbs into clothing, or try to put garments on the wrong way round?

Sequential Tasks. Test the patient's ability on tests of sequential hand movements, alternating tapping tests, alternating choice tasks, and alternating written sequences.

Other General Indications of Organic Cerebral Disease

Note the ability of the patient to sustain attention during the above tests. Did he fatigue unduly easily? Was he able to shift attention readily from one task to another? Was there perseveration in the use of words, in simple motor acts, or in response to commands? Observe for difficulties with abstract thinking; test for this by definition of concepts, e.g. difference between dwarf and child, or interpretation of proverbs.

Note and describe any evidence of lability of mood, euphoria, or indications of catastrophic reaction. Were emotional responses exaggerated, flattened, or lacking? Did he show impulsiveness, disinhibition, or over-familiarity? Did he appreciate his failings and show appropriate concern? Did he make use of evasions or excuses to cover up his defects?

Appendix B
Examination of the Mute or Apparently Inaccessible Patient

States of mutism, 'stupor', and apparent inaccessibility may be due to organic brain disease or functional psychiatric disorder. In all cases it is necessary to perform a detailed neurological examination and to assess the apparent level of conscious awareness (as outlined on page 15) before considering other aspects of the problem. It is also necessary to bear in mind the possibility of underlying metabolic disturbances, like uraemia or hypoglycaemia, and physical complications of stupor like hypotension and retention of urine. Finally it is important to remember that the patient's comprehension of remarks made in his presence may be good despite appearances to the contrary.

Stupor, Semi-coma and Hypersomnia. The definitions of these terms are not sufficiently precise to be used as the sole description of the phenomena they comprise. The following features should therefore be described separately:

To what extent can the patient dress, feed himself, and attend to matters of hygiene and elimination?

When aroused does he briefly become alert and verbally responsive?

Assess his response to graded stimulation (as outlined on page 16).

Are the eyes open or shut? If open, are they apparently watchful and do they follow moving objects? If shut, do they open in response to stimulation, is there resistance to passive opening?

Is the physical posture comfortable, constrained, awkward, or in any way bizarre? Does the patient resume a previous posture if moved or placed in an awkward or uncomfortable position? Are there any spontaneous movements or acts? If so, are movements meaningful; do acts display special meaning, possibly on a delusional basis or in response to possible hallucinatory experiences?

Is the facial expression constant or varying, alert or vacant, meaningful or unresponsive? Is there any physical or emotional reaction to what is said or done to the patient, or near him?

Examine the state of the musculature: is it relaxed or rigid? Is rigidity increased by passive movements? Test for negativism, waxy flexibility, automatic obedience, echopraxia. Note evidence of resistiveness, irritability, or defensive movements during examination.

In the neurological examination pay special attention to evidence of diencephalic or upper brain stem disturbance: observe equality and reactivity of pupils and note quality of respiration, look for evidence of long tract deficit in the limbs, test for conjugate reflex eye movements on passive head rotation.

After recovery examine for memory of events occurring during the abnormal phase, and for phantasies or other subjective experiences occurring at the time.

'**Mutism**' is a condition in which a person does not speak and does not make any attempt at spoken communication despite preservation of an adequate level of consciousness. It may sometimes be the only abnormality in otherwise normal behaviour. Is it elective, confined to some situations or in relation to some persons but not to others? Is the patient himself disturbed by it as shown by gesticulations or evidence of distress? Does he attempt to communicate by signs? When offered paper and pen can he communicate in writing?

Distinguish mutism from severe motor dysphasia, dysarthria, aphonia, poverty of speech or psychomotor retardation. Is partial vocalization preserved, are emotional ejaculations possible, can simple 'yes'/'no' answers be given? Test separately for ability to articulate (to whisper or make the lip movements of speech) and ability to phonate (to produce coarse vocalization or to hum). Can he cough? Does he speak very occasionally and briefly on restricted themes? Does he reply or signal responses to some questions but only after long delay?

A careful history from informants may sometimes enable distinctions to be made more readily than from examination alone.

Appendix C

The Gresham Ward Questionnaires
(For Elderly Patients)

These should be administered 3-4 days after admission and the patient's answers recorded verbatim for every question. (It is also vital for subsequent interpretation to record the date of examination.)

1 **General Orientation**

Where are you now?

What is this place called?

Where is it situated?

What day of the week is it today?

What month are we in?

What day of the month is it?

What is the year?

What time is it? (Allow 30 min. either way)

Maximum score 8. Score leniently for each question answered correctly.

2 Memory for Past Personal Events

Where were you born?

What year were you born? (exact year to score)

How old were you when you left school?

What year did you get married? (exact year to score)

(If unmarried, what year did you leave home?)

Where was your first employment?
(Rough indication such as 'a family in Clapham, a factory in Leeds, etc.' accepted.)

How many years since you were last employed?

(If still employed: How many years have you been in this job?)
('Not since the war' or 'not since I got married,' etc., accepted.)

When were you last in hospital?
(1 point either for exact year or 'three years ago', or something like that.)

When did your mother die?

How many jobs have you had?
(Rough estimate may do but not too marked deviation — such as 10 jobs if 15 in actual fact.)

When was your first child born? (exact year to score)
(If unmarried, use the birthday of a brother or sister.)

What was the name of the school you went to?

How old were you when you got married?
(If unmarried, how old were you when you left home?) Exact age for scoring.

Maximum score 12. Allow 1-2 years either way unless stated otherwise. If patient never had any employment, do not score *both* question 5 and 6.

3. Memory for Recent Personal Events

When were you admitted to this hospital? (Date and day of the week.)

How did you get here?
(Form of transport and route.)
1 point if either correct.
2 points if both correct.

Did anybody accompany you? Who?
1 point for correct answer.

Did you see another doctor before you came here?

1 point *only* if doctor's name given. (G.P.'s name does not score.)

Where did you see him and when?
1 point if either indicated.
2 points if both.
Exact name of place has to be given for scoring.
Re time — such statements as 'last month', etc., will do for scoring.

What is my name?
(Make sure you introduce yourself to patient once or twice during previous interviews.)
1 point only if exact.

When did I last see you?
1 point only if correct.

How many days ago did I take a blood test? (Or, did I take your blood pressure?)
1 point only if correct day is given.

Maximum score 11

4. Memory for General Events

Has anything important happened in the world recently?
(Score 1 point for important event, making allowances for patient's educational background.)

Who is on the Throne?

How many children has she got?

What are their names?
(1 point for number and another point if all 4 names correct.)

What is the name of the present Prime Minister?

Who was the Prime Minister before him?

What is the name of the President of the U.S.A.?

Who was the President before him?

When did the last war start/finish?
(2 points if both years correct. 1 point for one year correct.)

Nature of one recent strike, accident or national catastrophe. Where and when?
(2 points if both reasonably correct.)

Maximum score 12.